I0086931

ISBN-10: 0615563260
ISBN-13: 978-0615563268 (Little Vet)
Copyright © 2010 Lori Hehn. All rights reserved.
Little Vet is a trademark of Lori Hehn of
Hehn Veterinary, PLLC. All rights reserved.
First Printing 2011.

No portion of this book may be copied, retransmitted,
reposted, duplicated, or otherwise used without the
express written approval of the author. Any unauthorized
copying, reproduction, translation, or distribution of
any part of this material without permission by the
author is prohibited and against the law.

For more information visit us at www.LittleVet.com

Disclaimer: This book should not be used to diagnose
or treat any medical condition in animals.

RAZZ HAS SURGERY

A Little Vet™ Book

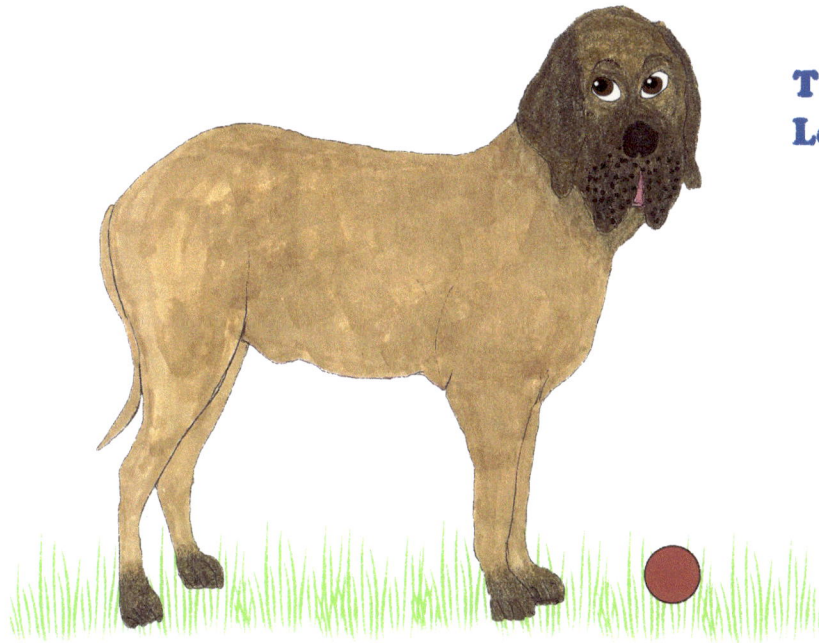

To: Gog
Love, Razz

Story by: Lori J. Hehn, DVM
Pictures by: Don E. Winters

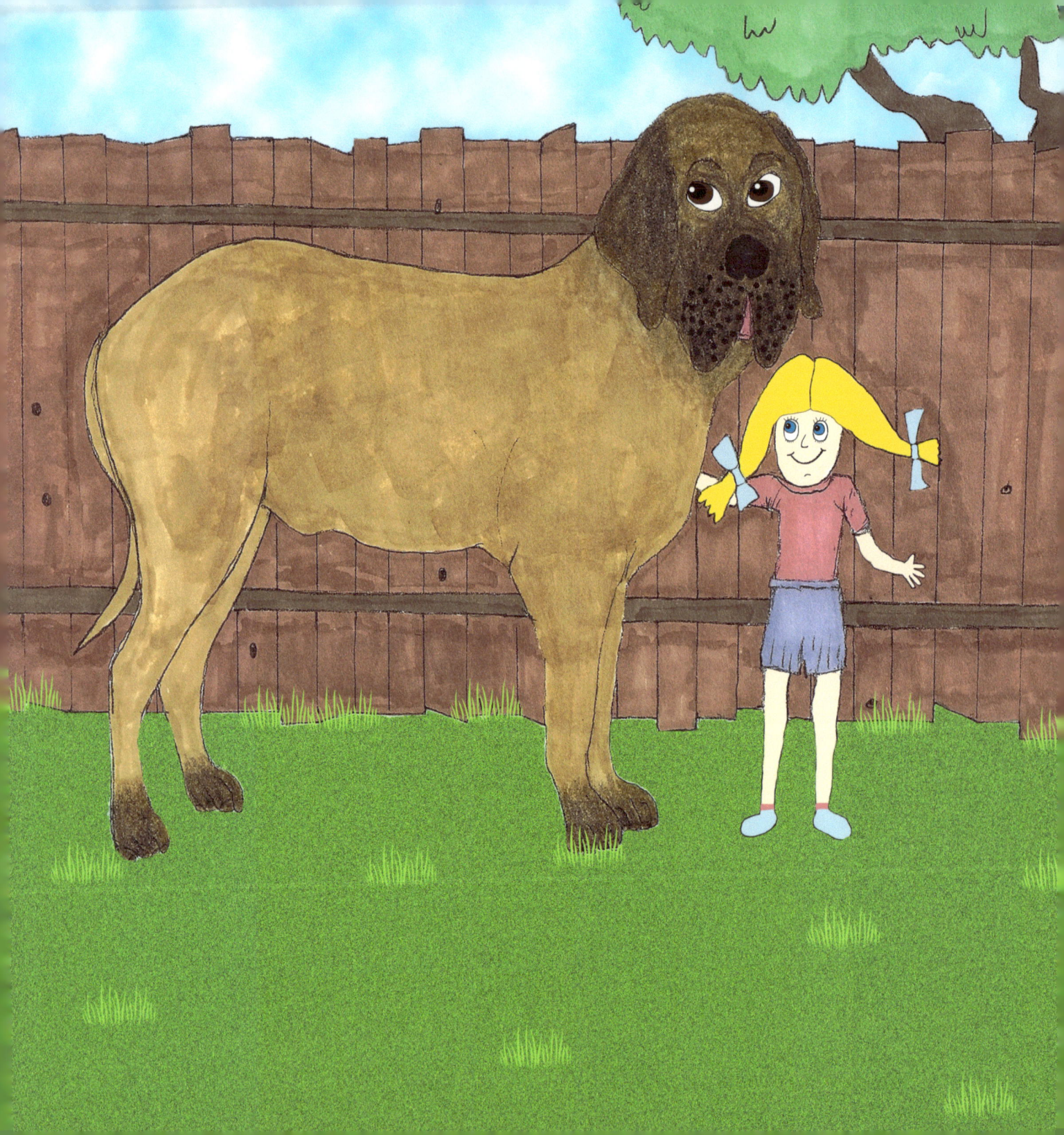

This is my dog Rascal T. Razzbone.

We call him Razz for short. He is an

English Mastiff!

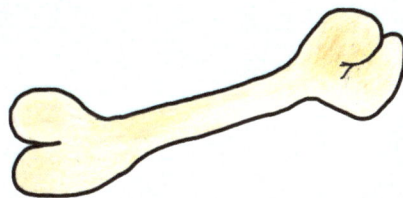

Razz may look big and tough, but he is really just a giant teddy bear!

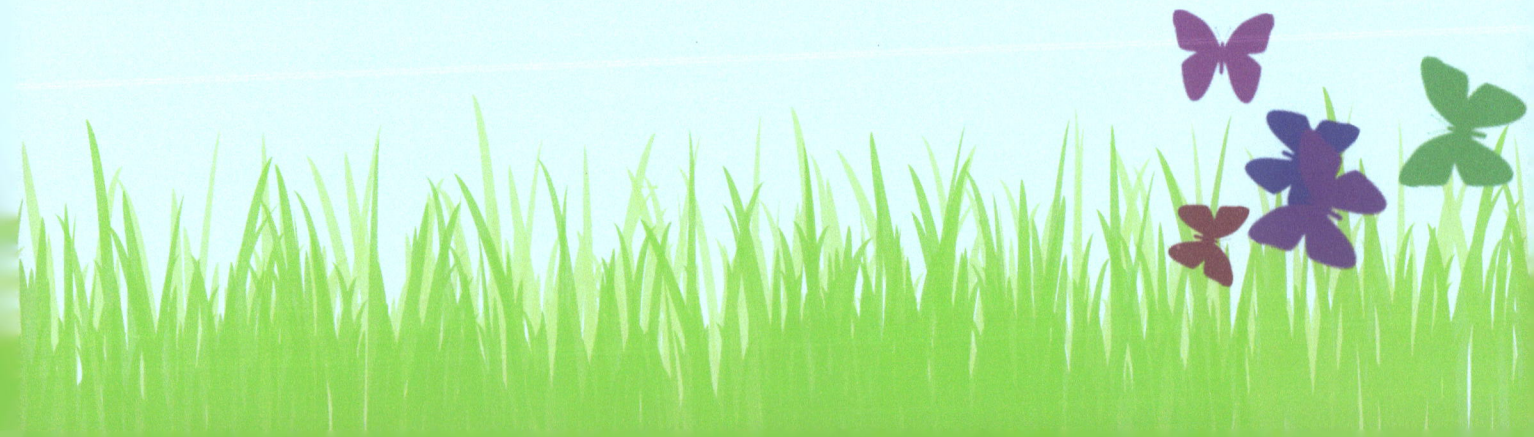

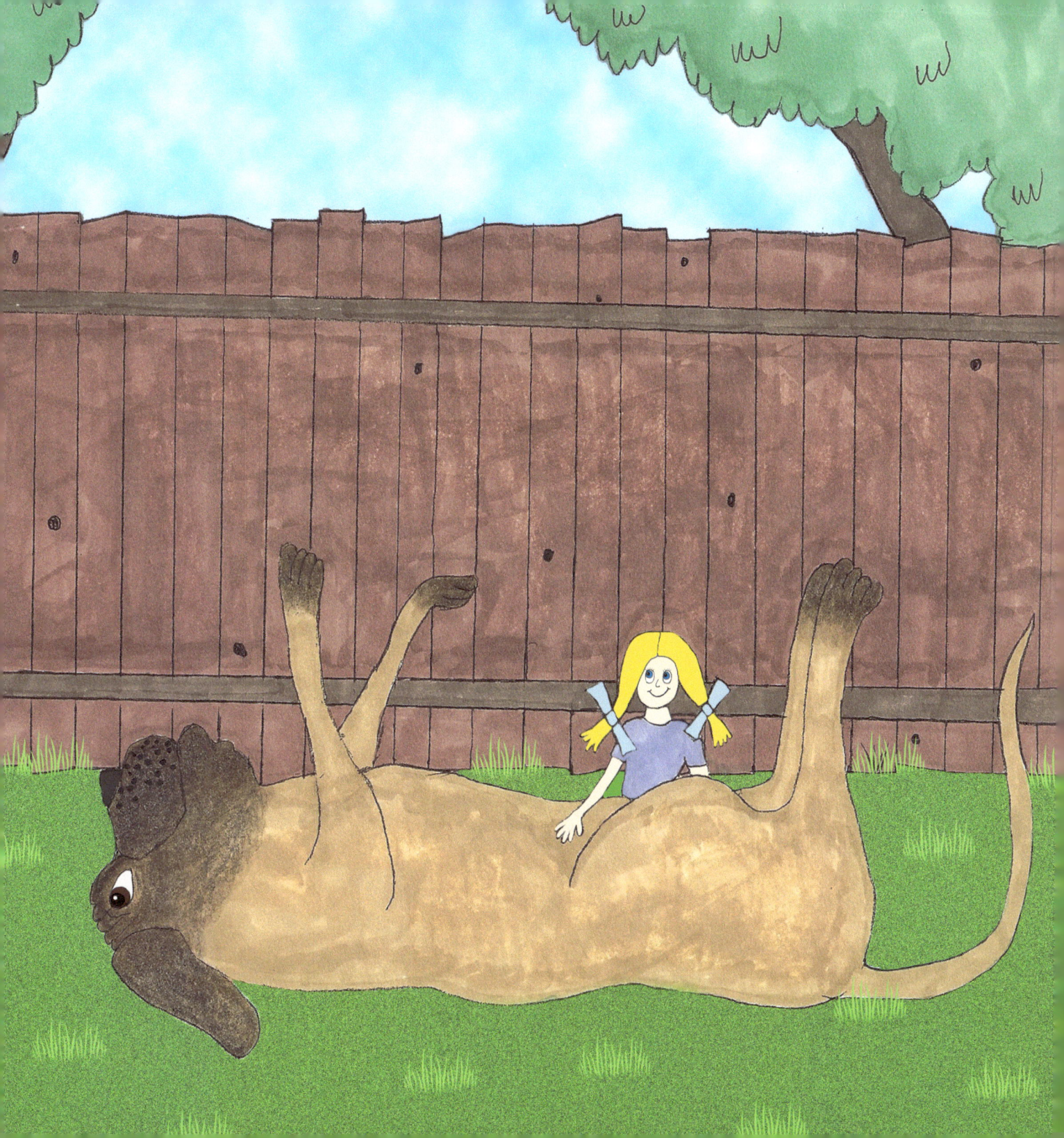

ANIMAL SHELTER

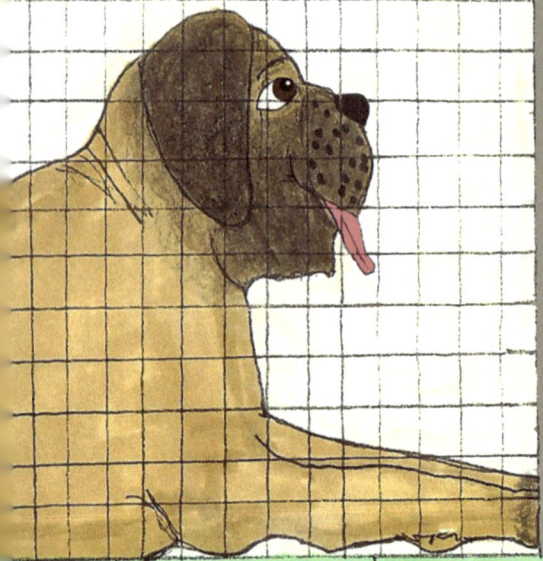

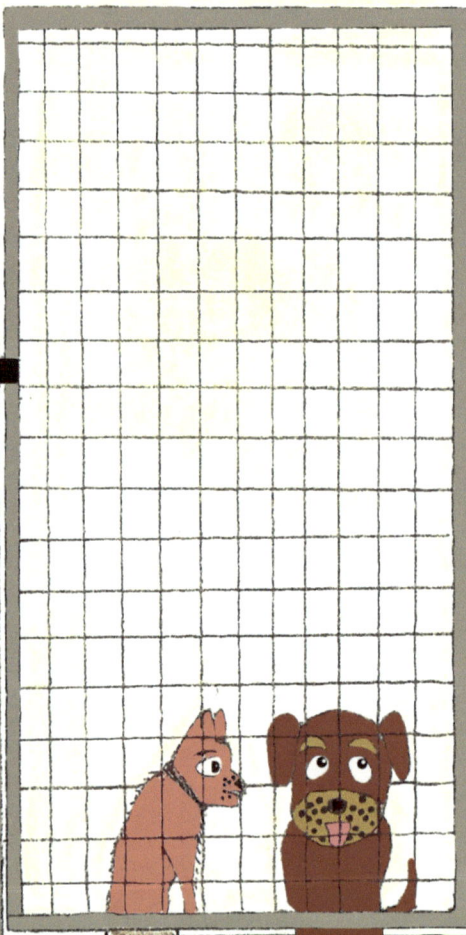

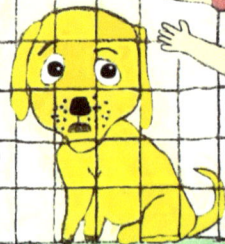

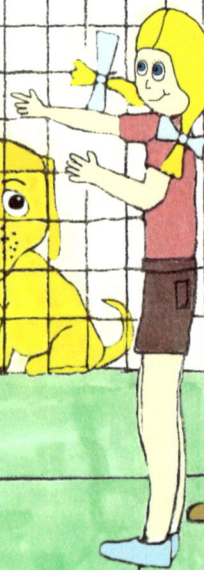

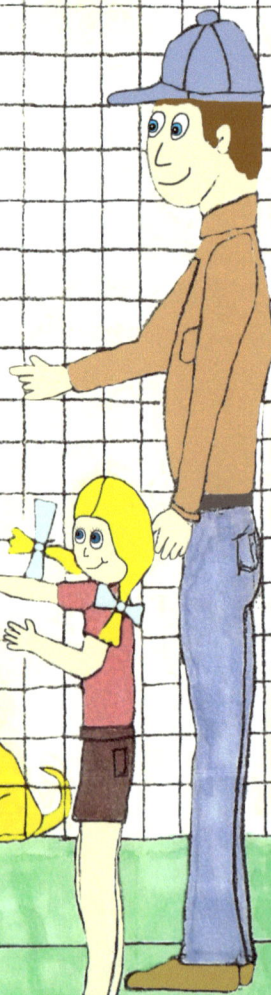

My family adopted Razz from the shelter because he needed a family to love him, and he did not have a home!

PLEASE ADOPT

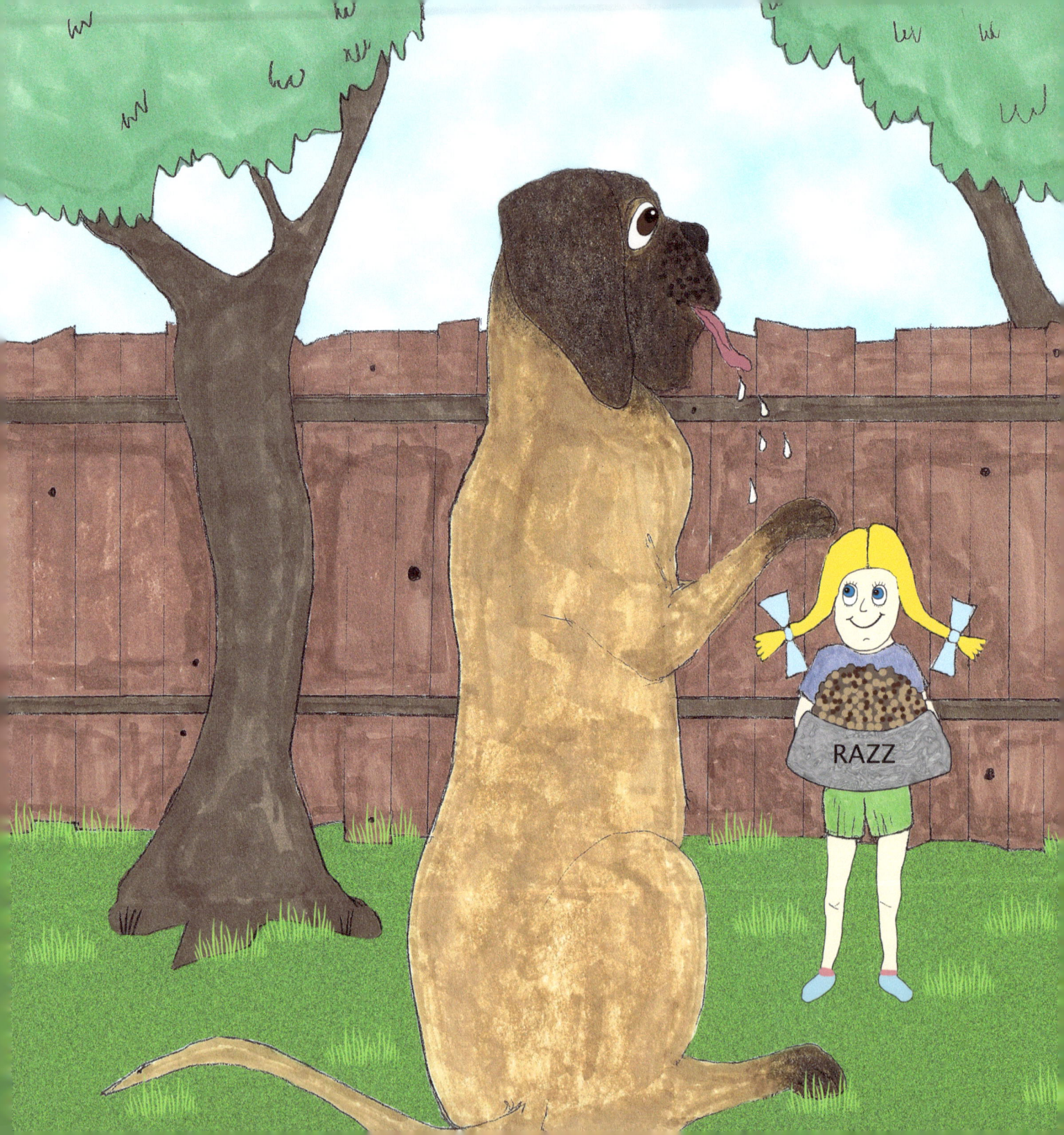

I am in charge of feeding
and watering Razz...

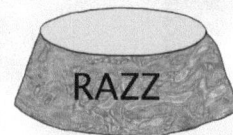

RAZZ

and scooping his poop,

which is a very BIG job!

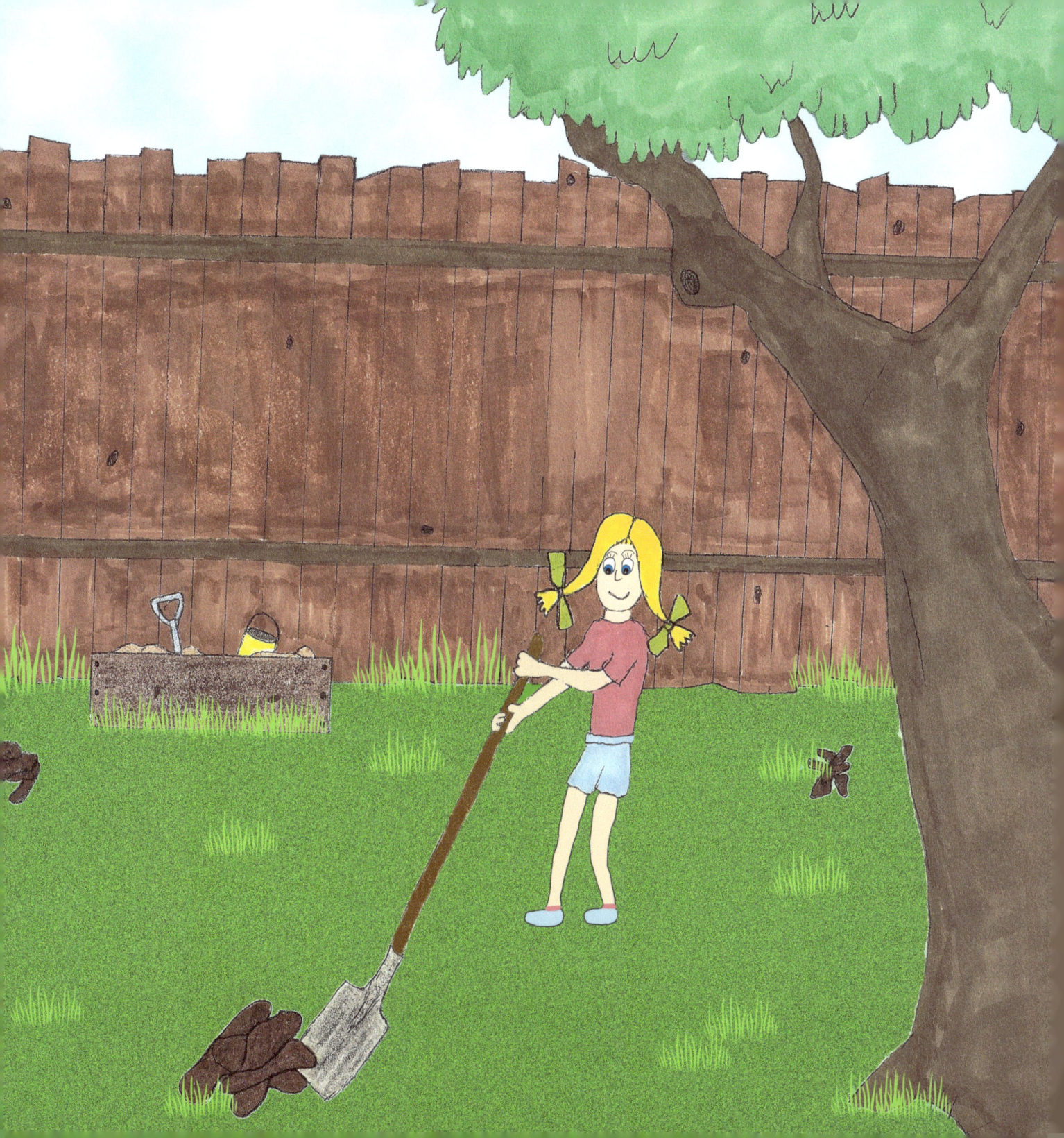

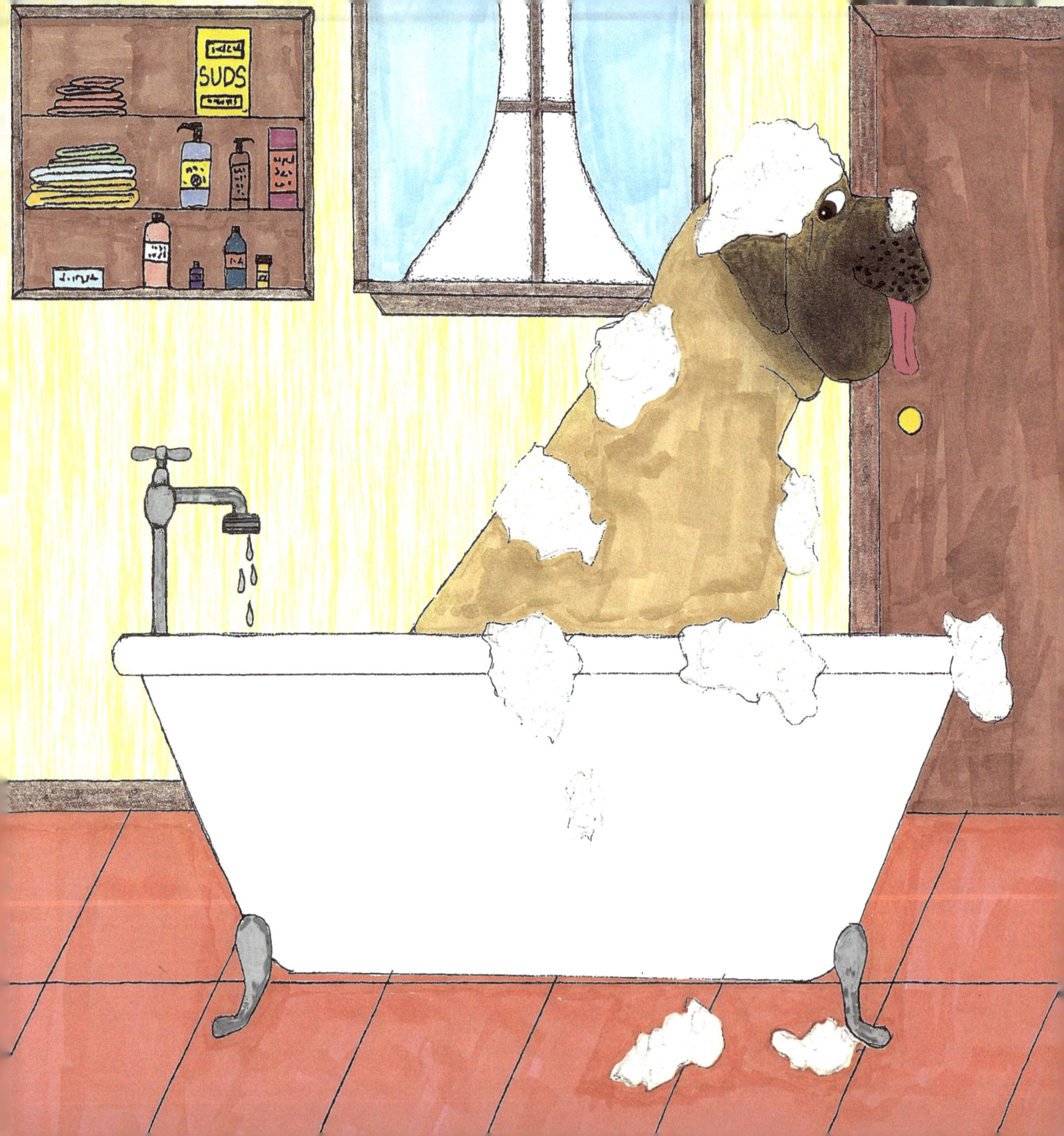

Razz weighs more than I do, so mom and dad have to help me give him a bath...

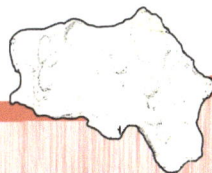

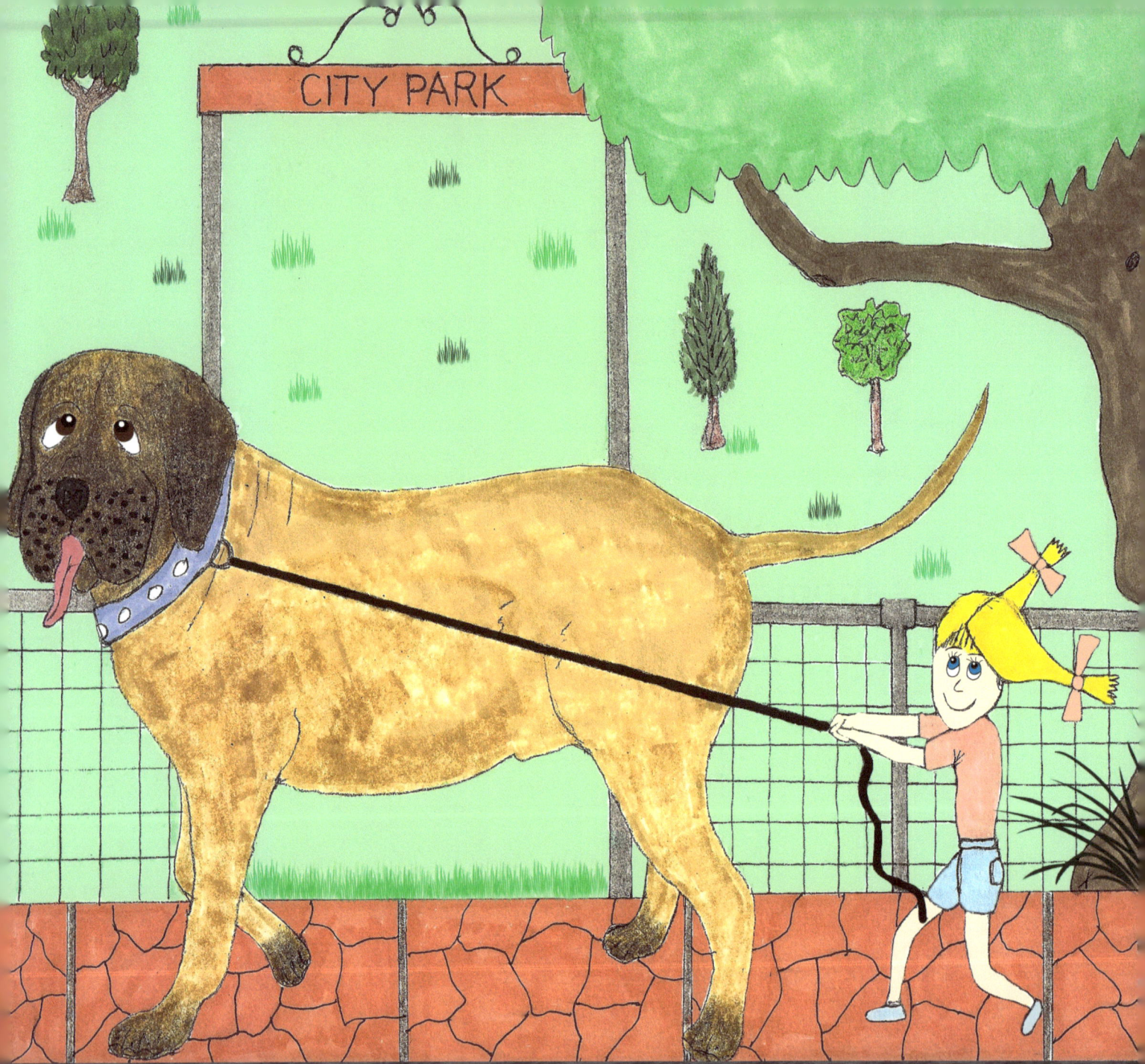

CITY PARK

and take him for his walks.
Otherwise, he takes me for a walk!

"Wait for me, Razz!"

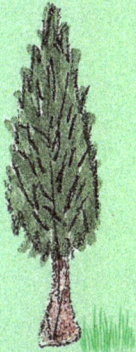

Razz has one bad habit.

He likes to eat things he shouldn't.

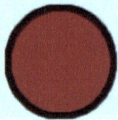

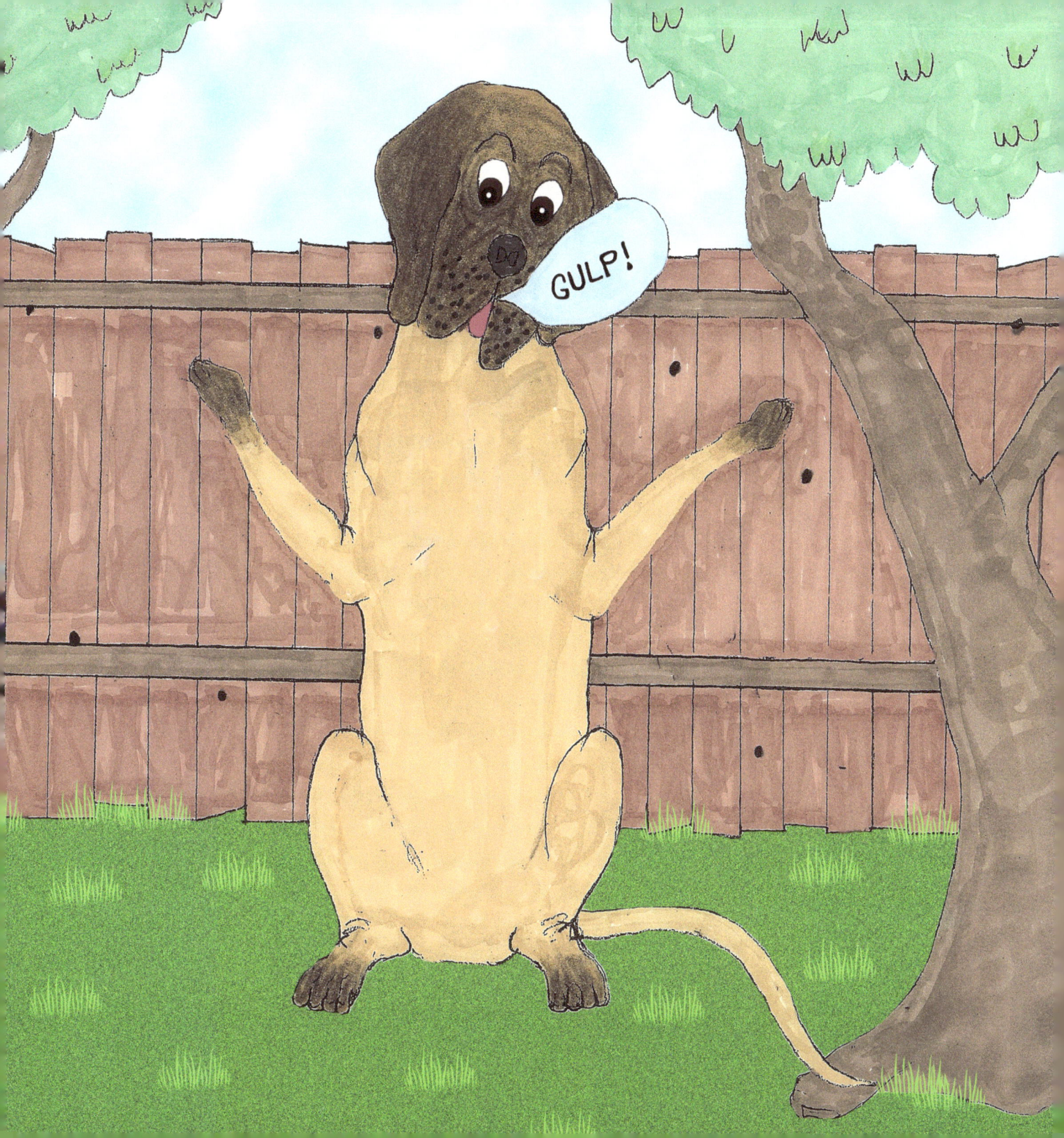

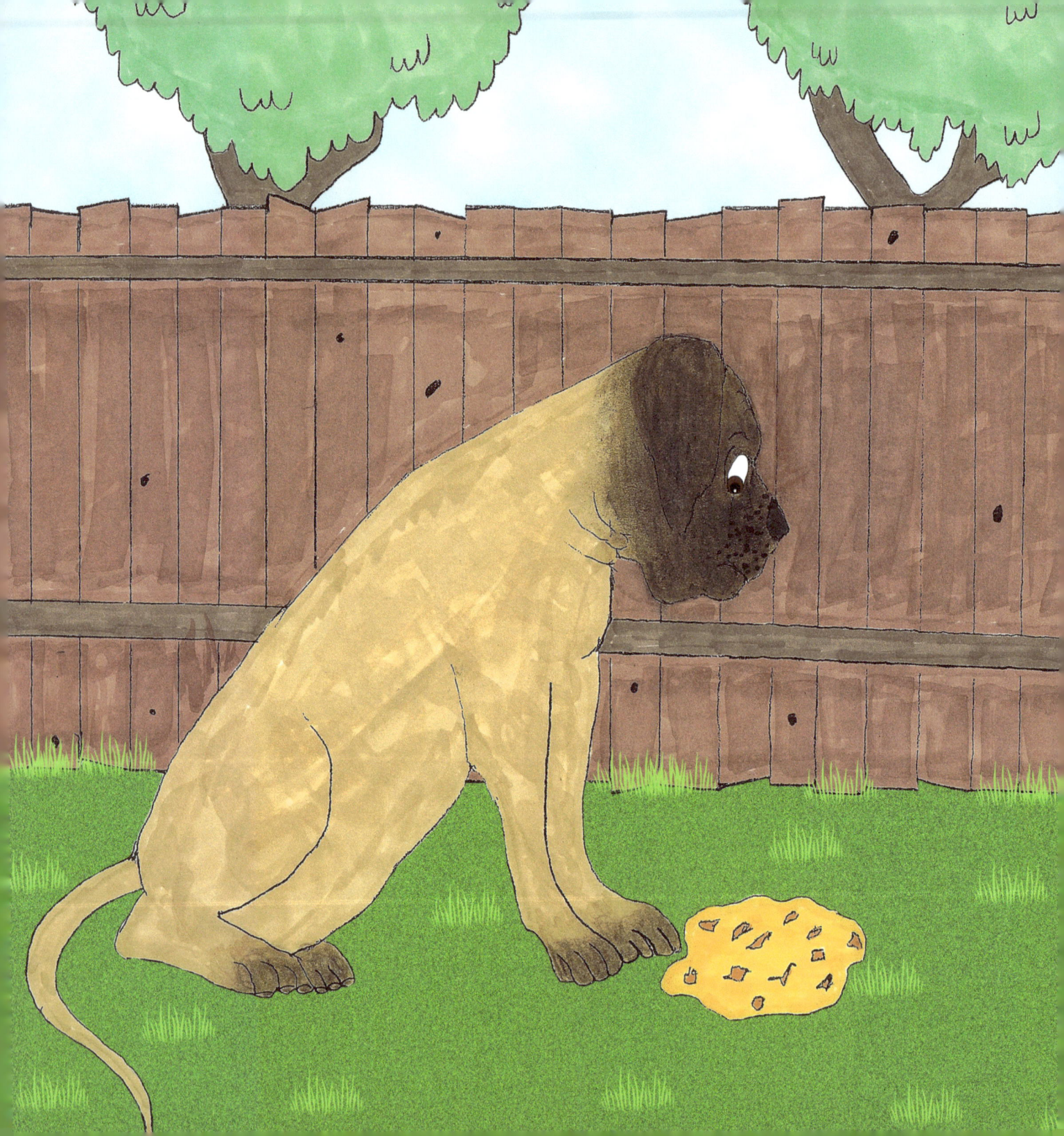

One day, Razz stopped eating.

He had no energy, and he started vomiting.

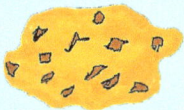

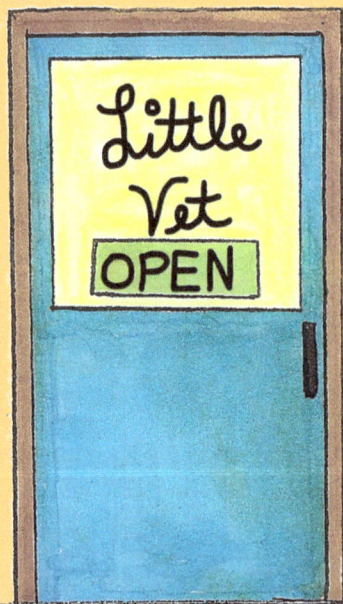

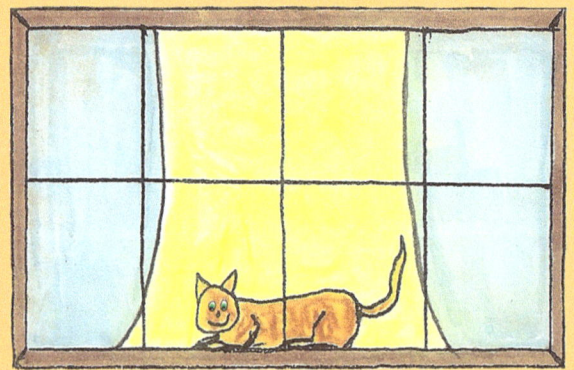

We took Razz to the veterinary hospital

to find out why hc was sick!

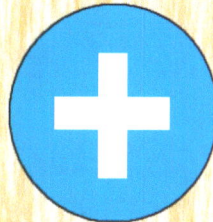

The vet took x-rays of his abdomen.

An x-ray is a picture of the inside of the body.

CAUTION: RADIATION
AUTHORIZED
PERSONNEL ONLY!

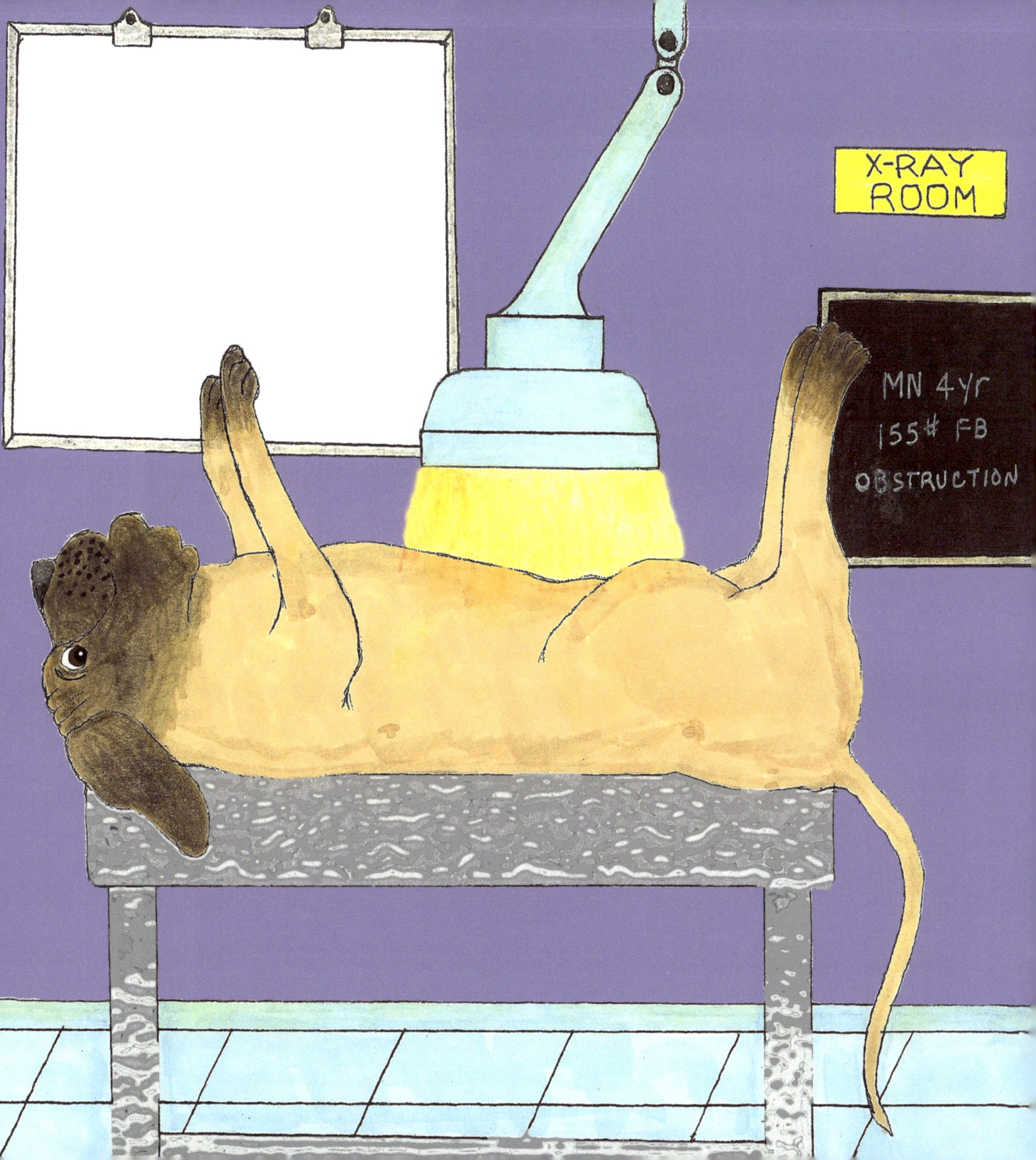

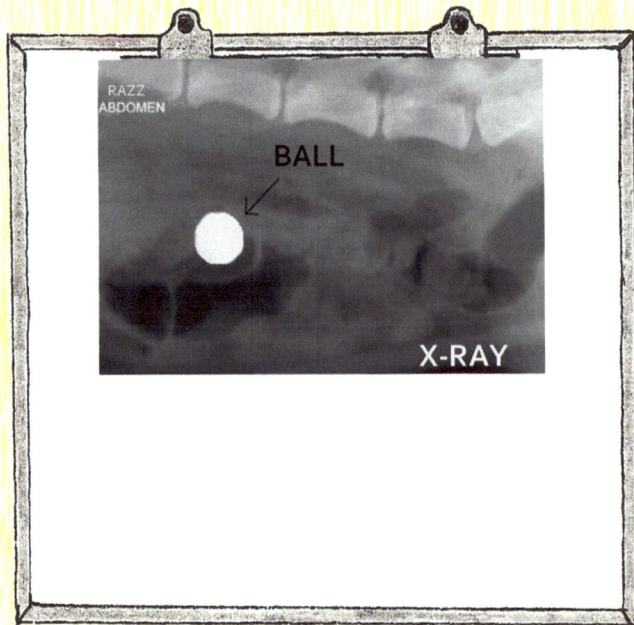

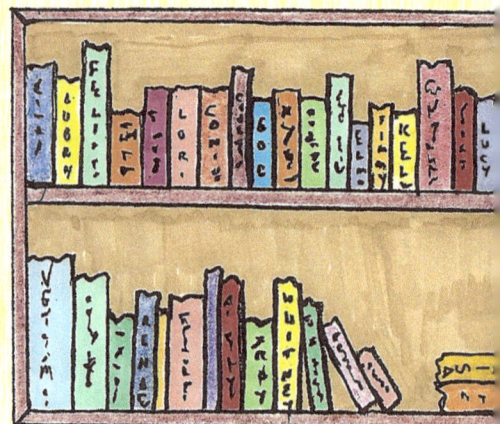

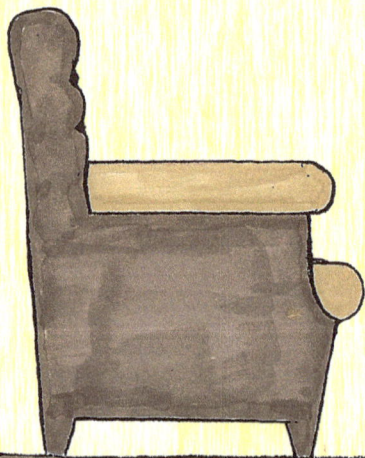

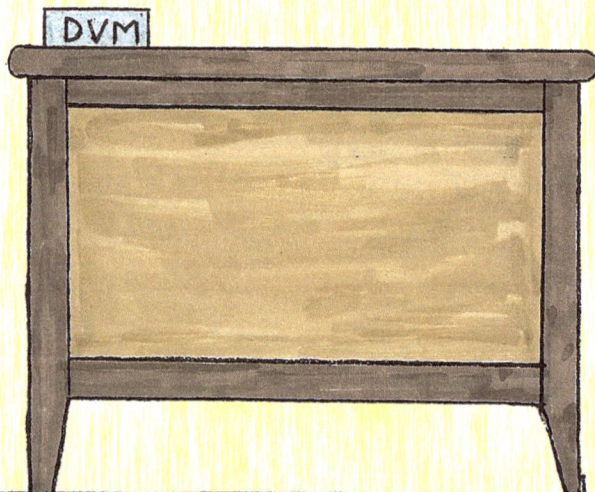

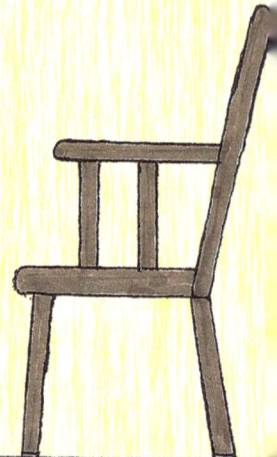

The x-ray showed a circle shape in his abdomen. "Uh oh!" the vet said. "It looks like Razz swallowed something that is stuck in his intestine!"

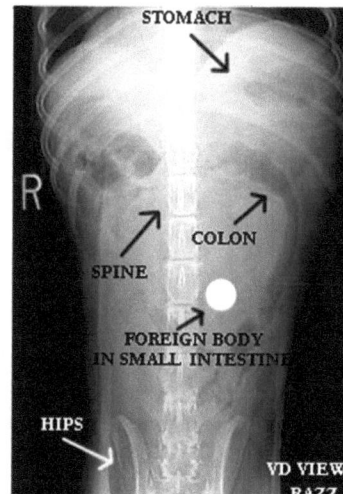

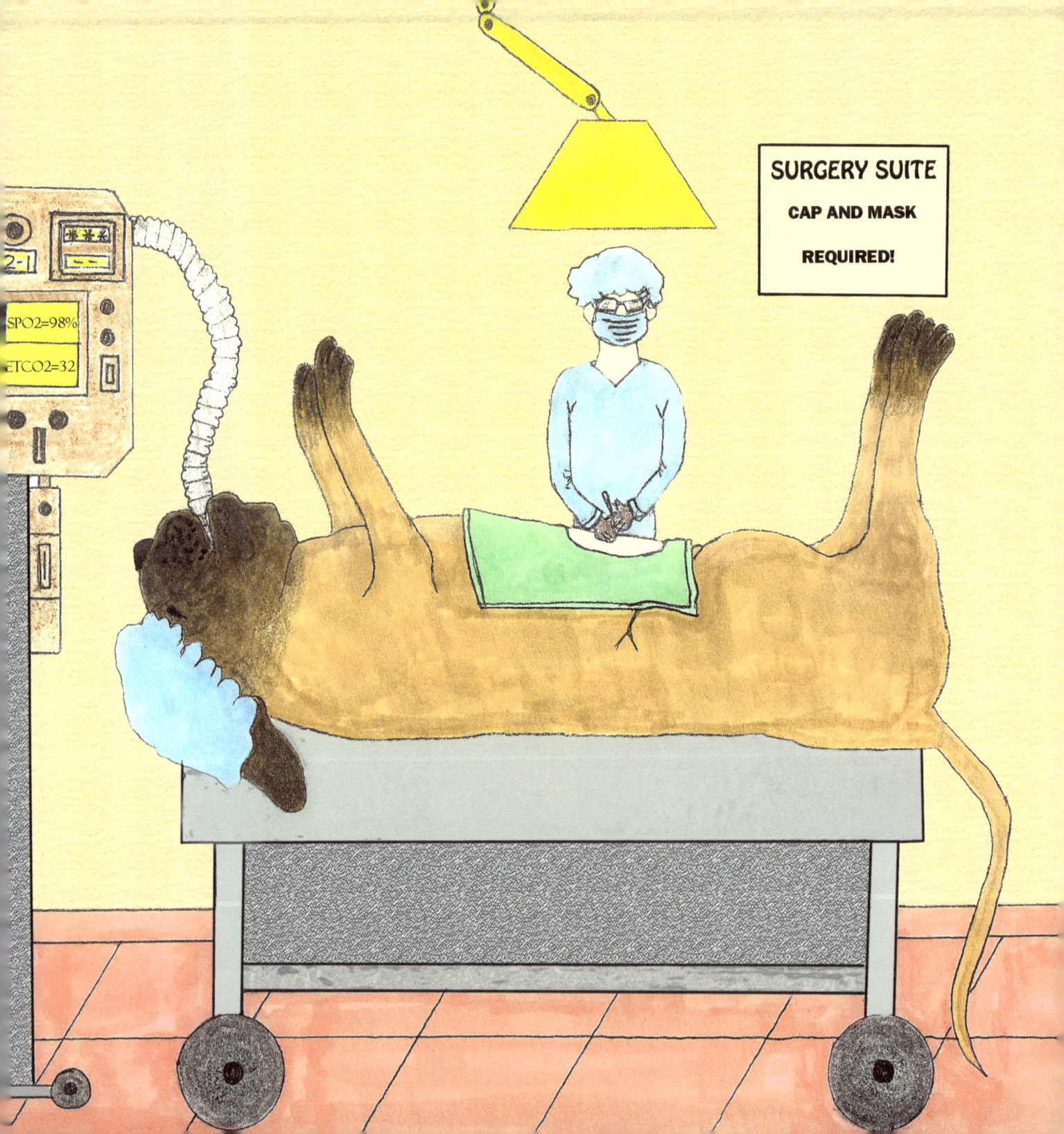

SURGERY SUITE

CAP AND MASK

REQUIRED!

SPO2=98%

ETCO2=32

The vet called the object a "foreign body". Razz needed surgery to remove it!

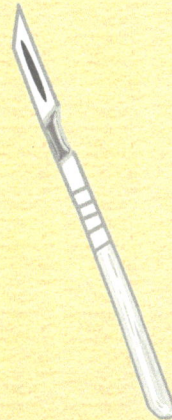

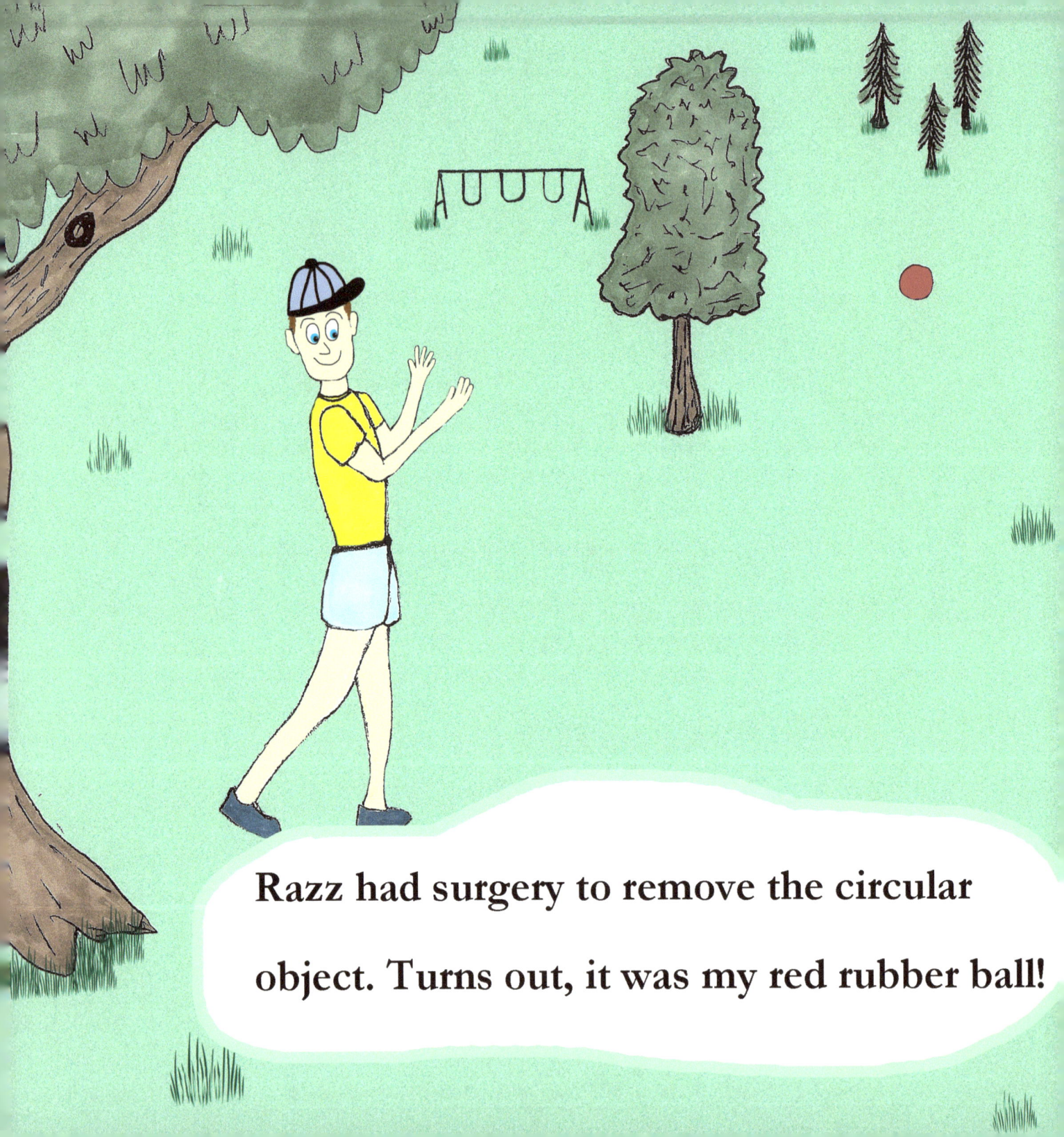

Razz had surgery to remove the circular object. Turns out, it was my red rubber ball!

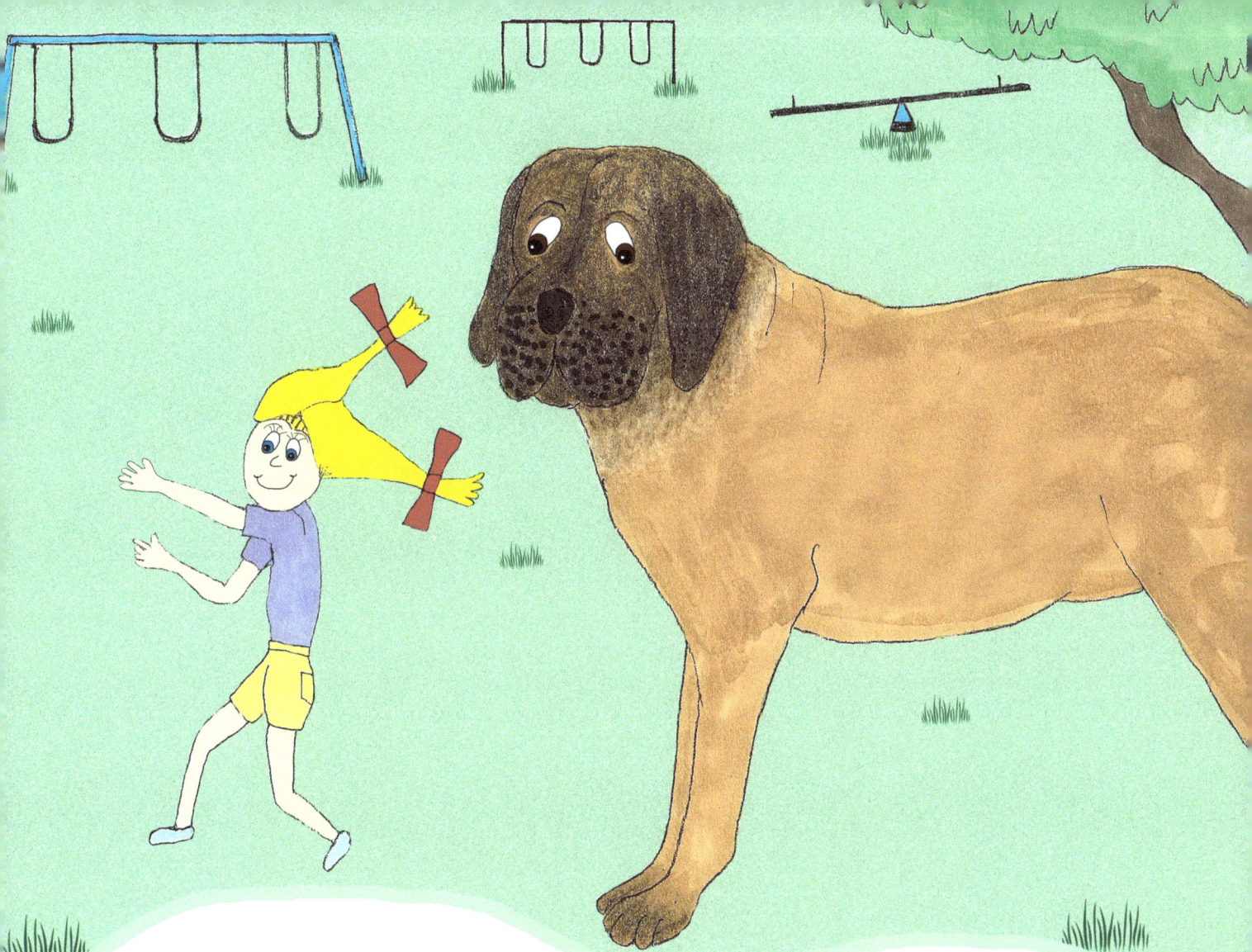

I was playing catch with my brother when it went missing!

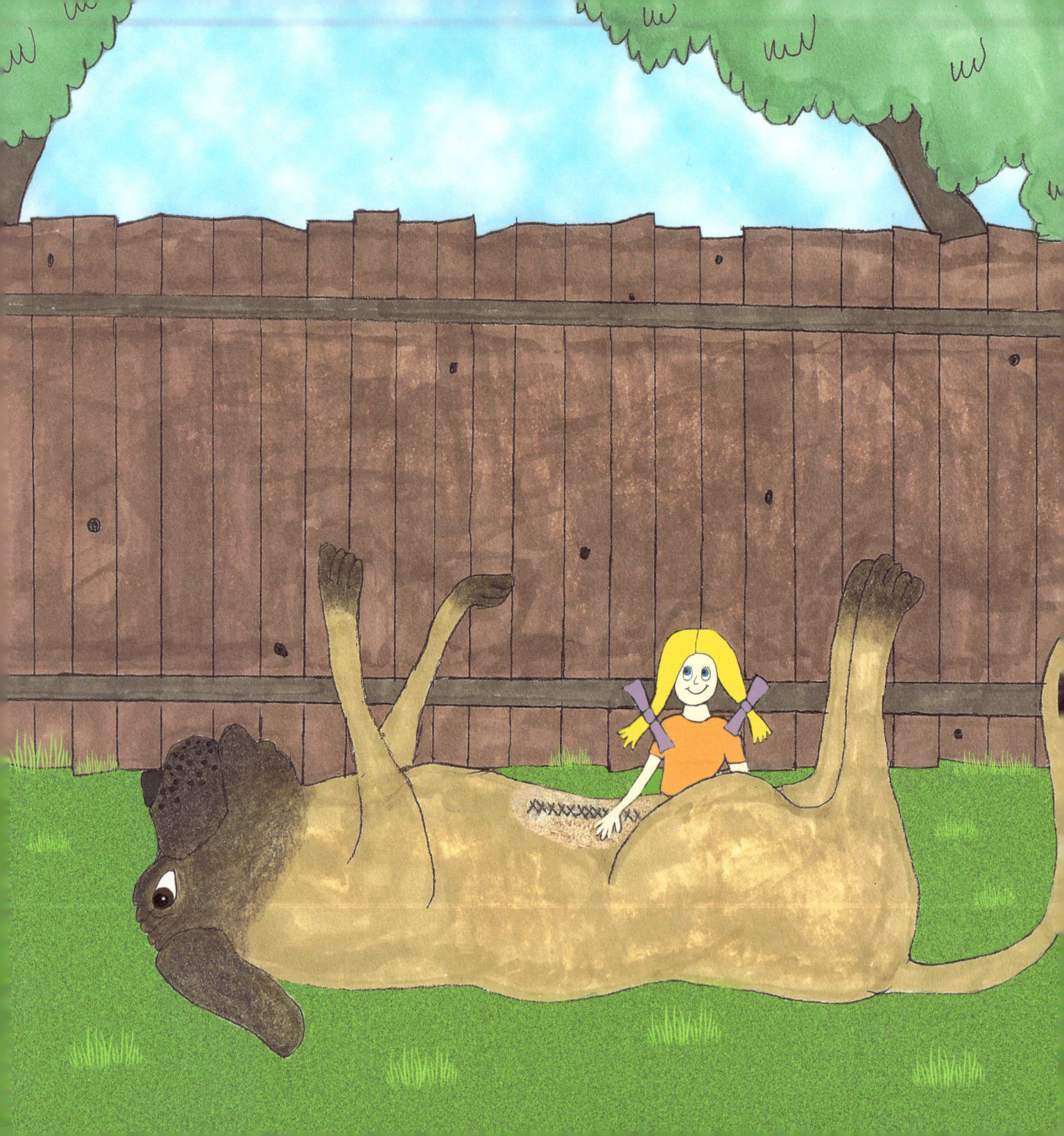

Razz was back to his old self again!

He had stitches in his belly after

his surgery.

My brother and I have to be extra careful, and always put our toys away so that Razz won't get them.

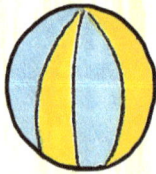

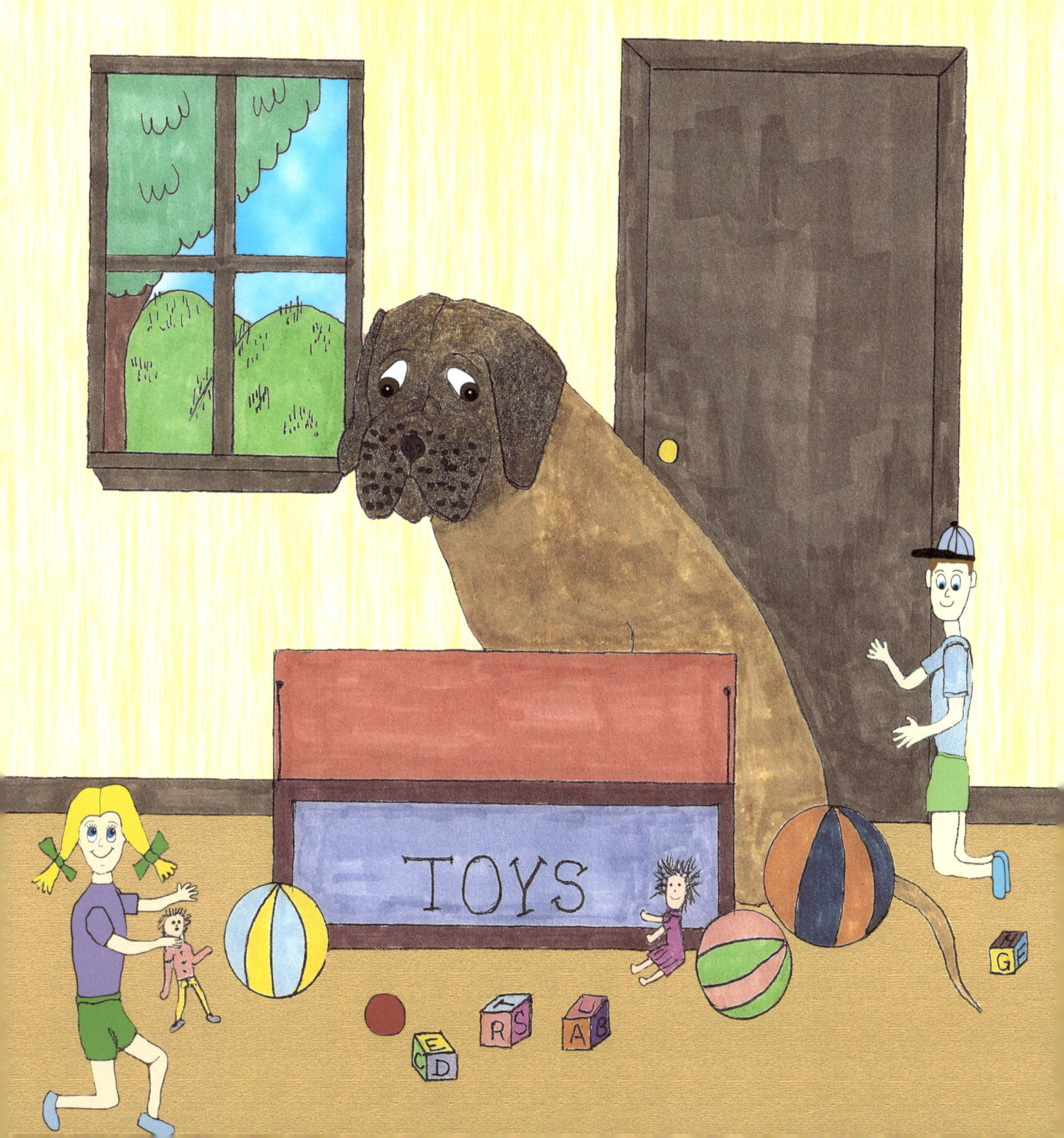

We love Razz and always want

him to be healthy!

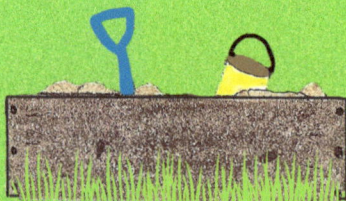

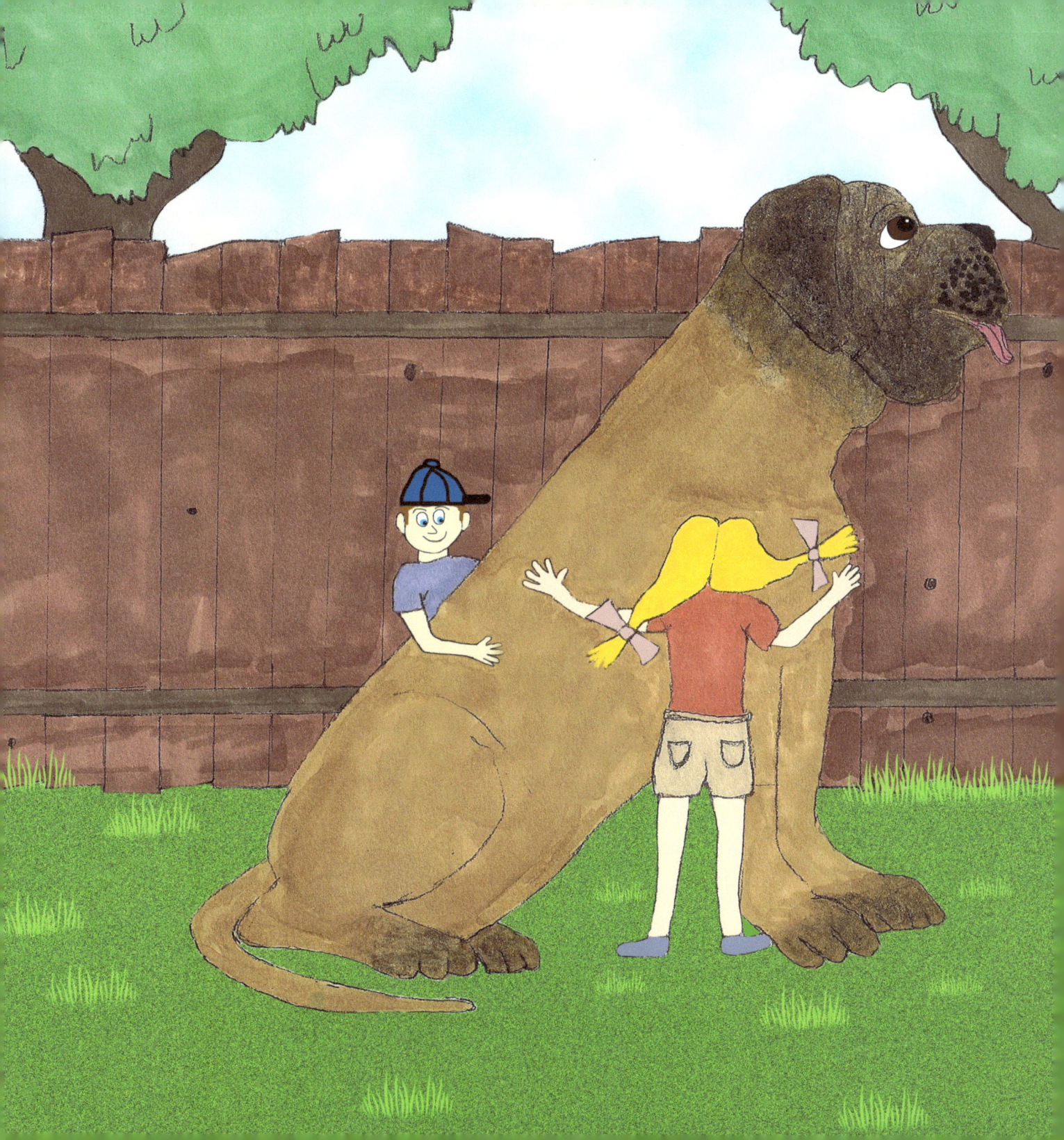

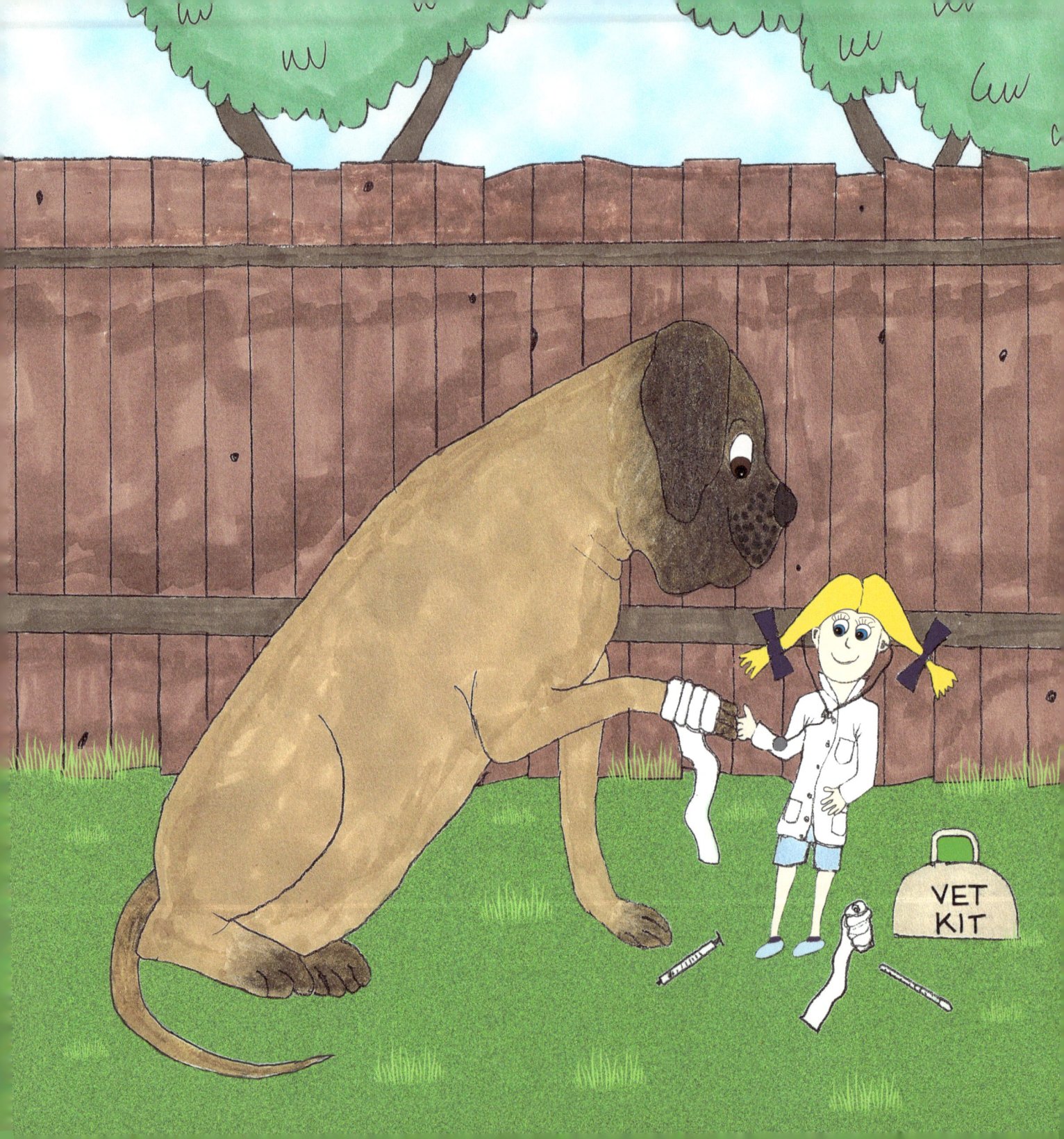

When I grow up, I want to be a veterinarian so I can help pets like Razz when they are sick!

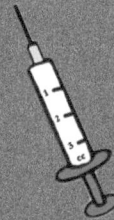

Glossary

Abdomen- the belly; The cavity between the chest and pelvis which holds the abdominal organs, including the liver, kidneys, stomach, intestine, spleen, pancreas, and bladder.

Adopt- giving a home to a pet that does not have one. This term is usually in reference to adopting a pet from a shelter or humane society.

Animal shelter- a place for animals to live that do not have a home. A shelter is usually a transient place that houses animals until they can find a family or place to live.

Foreign body- an object or extraneous matter that has entered the body.

Intestine- the longest part of the digestive tract is the small intestine. The small intestine absorbs nutrients from food into the body.

Surgery- a branch of medicine that treats diseases or injuries by incision or manipulation, especially with instruments (such as a scalpel).

Veterinarian- an animal doctor.

X-ray- a radiograph; a type of high energy radiation used to diagnose diseases by making pictures of the inside of the body.

About Little Vet™ Books
A note from the author:

My clients often tell me that when they were little they wanted to be a veterinarian when they grew up. I know my own children love stories about animals and love to pretend that they are veterinarians helping pets. Little Vet™ Books are designed for children who have the desire to learn more about animals and veterinary medicine.

The books in this series each include a different animal species. The books are narrated by the child in the book to whom the animal belongs. The child talks about the responsibilites of caring for his or her pet. The books introduce clinical signs of an illness seen manifesting in the character. The animal goes to the vet to be diagnosed and treated, and new simple medical terms are introduced.

These books are fun for children because they are able to help the vet make a diagnosis and follow a treatment plan, yet the books are simple to understand and fun to read.

I have enjoyed writing this series and hope you and your children will love reading Little Vet™ Books!

www.ingramcontent.com/pod-product-compliance
Lightning Source LLC
Chambersburg PA
CBHW041236040426
42445CB00004B/44